GLUCOSE SURGE

A Guide To Managing The Highs And Lows of Blood Sugar Levels

LINDA J. DUTTON

TABLE OF CONTENTS

INTRODUCTION

Regardless of age or physical condition, controlling blood sugar levels can be difficult. The effects of fluctuating glucose levels can be significant, ranging from weariness and headaches to more serious illnesses like diabetes, heart disease, and stroke.

It is acknowledged that dealing with diabetes and other illnesses with blood sugar can be daunting, difficult, and perplexing.

When you have diabetes, your body is unable to produce any insulin or enough insulin to transport sugar from the blood into your cells. High glucose or blood sugar levels result from this.

Glucose, often known as blood sugar, is a crucial part of our body's energy source.

It serves as our body's main source of energy for our muscles, brain, and other organs.

Since fluctuations can have a detrimental effect on our ability to function physically and mentally, maintaining balanced blood sugar levels is essential for general health and well-being.

If you have diabetes, controlling your blood glucose level is essential because the quantity of glucose varies throughout the day. This is due to the possibility of long-term problems from high blood sugar levels.

Our blood sugar levels can be impacted by a variety of factors, including nutrition, exercise, and medical problems, making it difficult to maintain stable glucose levels throughout the day.

The ins and outs of controlling blood sugar will be covered, along with advice on how to keep levels stable and spot high and low blood sugar warning signs.

You will learn about how blood sugar levels function, the many types of diabetes, how to monitor blood sugar levels, meal planning, ideal exercise, and more with the help of brief and clear explanations and useful advice.

Read on for a thorough explanation of blood sugar management whether you're managing diabetes, a healthcare professional, a caregiver, someone who wants to recover control over their blood sugar levels, or you simply wish to enhance your health.

Glucose Surge

UNDERSTANDING BLOOD GLUCOSE LEVELS

What Exactly Is Glucose?

The word glucose is derived from the Greek word for *"sweet."* Your body requires this particular sort of sugar, which it obtains from the meals you consume, to provide energy for cell function.

The most prevalent monosaccharide, a type of carbohydrate, is often glucose. One of the three macronutrients your body needs for energy, along with fat and protein, or amino acids, carbohydrates are a compound of hydrogen, carbon, and oxygen.

Glucose is primarily produced by plants and the majority of algae during photosynthesis from water and carbon dioxide with the help of solar energy, where it is used to create cellulose in cell walls.

The control of glucose metabolism is crucial. It is known as blood glucose or blood sugar when it goes through your bloodstream to your cells.

The main type of sugar in your blood is called blood glucose, or blood sugar. The majority of your meal is converted by your body into glucose, which is then released into your bloodstream. Your pancreas releases insulin when your blood glucose levels rise. Insulin transfers glucose from the bloodstream into cells for usage as fuel and storage.

Where Does Your Body Get Its Glucose From?

The most typical monosaccharide present in nature is glucose. It is produced in plants by photosynthesis. In some plants, chains of glucose are stored. We refer to these chains as starch. Corn, potatoes, rice, and wheat are examples of common foods that include starch. In order to produce dextrose, glucose, maltodextrins, polyols, and high fructose corn syrup, which are utilized as ingredients in the creation of several foods, beverages, dressings, and sauces, starch is professionally separated from these complete food sources. Honey and dried fruits including dates, apricots, raisins, currants, cranberries, and prunes are the most potent whole-food sources of glucose monosaccharides.

While you are eating, food travels via your esophagus from your mouth to your stomach. There, enzymes and acids break it down into minute particles. Glucose is released during that procedure. It moves into your intestines, where it will be absorbed. It then enters your bloodstream from there. Once in circulation, insulin aids in the delivery of glucose to your cells.

However, glucose doesn't always have to come from food and drink right away. The body will occasionally produce glucose to make sure we always have plenty. By dissolving glycogen to release the glucose it contains, this can be accomplished.

Between meals or during times of vigorous exercise, glycogen is broken down.

The liver is primarily responsible for the gluconeogenesis process, which enables the body to produce glucose from non-carbohydrate sources.

When glycogen stores are depleted and glucose consumption is inadequate or nonexistent, as is the case during starvation or extended fasting, gluconeogenesis takes place.

Ideally, your body uses glucose several times per day. When you eat, it immediately gets to work breaking down glucose and other carbohydrates. The pancreas then assists enzymes as they start to break them down. Your body's ability to process glucose depends on the pancreas, which makes hormones like insulin.

The term "blood sugar level," "blood sugar concentration," "blood glucose level," or "glycemia" refers to the amount of concentrated glucose in the blood.

As part of maintaining metabolic homeostasis, the body strictly controls blood glucose levels.

Blood glucose levels are moderately controlled by the body so that there is just enough of it to power the cells without becoming too high. To sustain essential body activities, the inside environment of the blood must remain constant.

Throughout the day, blood glucose levels can fluctuate. After a meal, levels rise for about an hour before dropping down. They are at the lowest level right before the morning meal. Your blood glucose levels increase after eating, causing the beta cells to produce insulin into the bloodstream.

Insulin functions as a key to open the doors for glucose to enter the muscle, fat, and liver cells.

Almost all of the cells in your body are fuelled by glucose, lipids, and amino acids (protein's components).

However, it serves as your brain's primary source of fuel. It is necessary for information processing by the nerve cells and chemical messengers there. Without it, your brain cannot function properly.

A few hours after your last meal, your blood glucose level drops. As a result, your pancreas ceases to produce insulin.

Alpha cells of the pancreas begin to create glucagon, a novel hormone. It directs the liver to dissolve stored glycogen to convert it to glucose.

It then enters your bloodstream to replenish your supplies till you can eat again.

When your blood glucose falls, your liver can also produce its glucose by combining waste materials, amino acids, and lipids.

THE IMPACT OF BLOOD GLUCOSE LEVELS ON THE BODY

As glucose is constantly being given to cells and replaced, a specific glucose molecule is never in the bloodstream for very long. This homeostatic threshold, which is between around 70 mg/dL and 100 mg/dL, requires remarkable coordination of a variety of physiological systems.

Insulin and glucagon fight it out to either eliminate glucose from the circulation (insulin) or add extra from storage (glucagon) in a never-ending tug of war.

Our activities play a significant role in our blood sugar levels changing throughout the day. My body can be flooded with glucose if I choose to consume a huge bowl of sugary cereal.

With other metabolites, this apparent cause and effect are less pronounced.

Glucose has a rather immediate impact on us. You can have normal, high, or low glucose levels. It's critical to be aware of your glucose level so that it can be managed and the risk of damage reduced.

Normal Blood Glucose Level

The ideal blood glucose levels differ depending on a person's age, the drugs they take, their diabetes status and duration of diabetes, as well as any other illnesses that may affect blood sugar.

Fasting blood glucose (in between meals):
The normal range for fasting blood sugar is 70 to 100 mg/dL.

Preprandial glucose (before a meal): Blood sugar levels before eating should be between 80 and 130 milligrams per deciliter (mg/dL) for adults who are not pregnant, less than 95 mg/dL for pregnant women with gestational diabetes, and 70 mg/dL to 95 mg/dL for pregnant women with pre-existing type 1 or type 2 diabetes.

Postprandial glucose (1-2 hours after eating): Less than 180 mg/dL is the desired level for adult non-pregnant individuals. The goal for those with gestational diabetes is less than 140 mg/dL after one hour and fewer than 120 mg/dL at two hours following a meal. One hour after a meal, pregnant women with type 1 or type 2 diabetes should have levels of 110 mg/dL to 140 mg/dL, and two hours after a meal, they should be 100 mg/dL to 120 mg/dL.

Before physical activity: Exercise can deplete energy and induce low blood sugar levels. In general, you should aim for a range of 126 mg/dL to 180 mg/dL before activity.

If your reading is less than 100 mg/dL after exercise, try consuming 15 to 20 grams of carbs to boost your blood sugar.

Check your blood sugar after 15 minutes, and if it is still less than 100 mg/dL, consume another 15-gram carbohydrate serving.

Repeat every 15 minutes until you reach the minimum level of 100 mg/dL.17 This is known as the 15-15 rule.

In addition to nutrition, activity, and how well your body creates and uses insulin, there are several other factors that may affect glucose levels, including:

1. Consumption of coffee: You may become especially sensitive to caffeine's ability to raise blood sugar levels even if you drink black coffee.

2. Stress level: Stress and concern in excess may raise blood sugar levels.

3. Getting a sunburn: Stress caused by sunburn pain may raise blood sugar levels.

4. Skipping meals: If you skip breakfast, your blood sugar levels after lunch and dinner may increase.

5. Medications: Certain drugs and nasal sprays may cause your liver to produce more glucose or stop the production of insulin.

6. The time of the day: Your body has a harder time controlling glucose as the day goes on. Early in the morning, the hormone surge may result in a blood sugar increase.

7. Less consumption of water

8. Lack of sleep

9. Some conditions, such as gum disease

Hypoglycemia

When a glucose level falls below 70 mg/dL, it is considered too low. This is also known as hypoglycemia, and it can be fatal. Certain diabetes drugs can cause hypoglycemia if you take more than the recommended dosage. It may also occur if you consume fewer calories than your daily requirements or exercise for a longer or more intense period than usual. It can happen to persons who don't have diabetes in some cases.

Consuming a meal or drinking juice may assist in raising glucose levels. Your doctor may be able to assist you in developing a plan for when your glucose level dips too low (or too high), which may include keeping glucose supplements on hand. Hypoglycemia can be fatal if untreated. When this happens, you may require immediate treatment.

When your blood sugar drops, there are symptoms to look out for. These consist of:

1. **Unusual Heartbeat**: Your heart rate may increase and it could feel like it skips a beat due to the hormones that assist boost blood sugar levels when they are too low. This is referred to as arrhythmia. Most frequently, the dip in glucose is brought on by medications used to treat diabetes.

2. **Hunger**: Even after eating, experiencing sudden, acute hunger may indicate that your body isn't properly converting food to blood sugar. It may also result from illness or some medications.

3. **Shakiness**: Your central nervous system, which regulates your movements, may become unbalanced by low blood sugar. Your body responds by releasing hormones to help your levels return to normal, such as adrenaline.

The same substances, however, may also cause trembling or shaking in your hands and other body parts.

4. **Dizziness**: Your brain cells require glucose for effective operation. When they run out, you might begin to feel weak, exhausted, and lightheaded. A headache could also be present.

5. **Fatigue**: Using insulin to decrease high blood sugar levels is one option if you have diabetes. However, if you consume too much, your body may be unable to swiftly replenish the glucose that is removed. You're exhausted as a result. Your tank may be drained by other illnesses and medications that disrupt this cycle.

6. **Sweating**: When your blood sugar drops too low, your body releases hormones that increase it while also making you sweat a lot.

When your glucose levels drop too low, it's frequently one of the first things you notice.

7. **Confusion**: You begin to become disoriented when your blood sugar levels drop drastically. Your words can become slurred, and you might lose track of your whereabouts. You might not even be aware that you're acting weirdly at times because it happens so quickly. In extreme circumstances, you can experience a seizure or coma.

Hyperglycemia

The term "hyperglycemia" refers to a high blood sugar level. This could occur if your body is not producing enough insulin or is not able to utilize it effectively.

Blood glucose levels above 130 mg/dL before a meal are regarded by the ADA (American Diabetes Association) as being above the target range.

Approximately one to two hours after eating, the ADA (American Diabetes Association) recommends a goal range of 180 mg/dL.
There are other reasons for hyperglycemia than uncontrolled diabetes. For instance, anxiety and stress may cause diabetes to be poorly managed. And this may result in more glucose in the blood. The following are some signs of hyperglycemia to watch out for:

1. **Dry Mouth**: As your body removes fluid from your mouth, it may become dry and develop cracks at the corners. Infection is more common when you spit less and have higher blood sugar levels. More water consumption or chewing sugar-free gum may be beneficial.

2. **Increased thirst**: Your body absorbs water from its own tissues to flush out the additional sugar. A switch in your brain flips to notify you that you're thirsty so you'll drink more fluid because you need

that fluid to create energy, transmit nutrients, and get rid of waste.

3. **Frequent urination**: Processing all of the excess sugar in your blood puts a lot of strain on your kidneys. Your body eliminates it, along with the water that it requires, when they are unable to keep up.

4. **Skin Issues**: To eliminate additional blood sugar, your body draws water from many sources. That could result in dry, itchy, cracked skin, particularly on your hands, feet, elbows, and legs. Elevated glucose levels have the potential to impair the neurological system over time. The term for this is diabetic neuropathy. You might find it more difficult to feel cuts, wounds, or infections as a result.

Without treatment, they may worsen and result in the loss of a foot, a toe, or perhaps a portion of your leg.

5. **Vision Problems**: Focusing may be made more challenging by your body's tendency to remove fluid from your eye lenses. Additionally, having high blood sugar might harm the retinal blood vessels in your eyes. That may result in permanent visual loss or perhaps total blindness.

What Happens If Your Blood Glucose Levels Are Not Controlled?

Poor glucose management over time has a harmful impact on your health. When your blood sugar levels are consistently high, you could start to notice the following:

- Numbness and tingling in the hands and feet
- Blindness
- Heart disease
- Joint pains
- Skin infections
- Severe dehydration
- Coma

Diabetes ketoacidosis and hyperglycemic hyperosmolar syndrome are two further serious complications. Both are diabetes-related issues. With repeated instances of low blood sugar, a condition called hypoglycemia unawareness may develop. It makes you less aware of low blood glucose symptoms until it is really low. If it drops too low, you might notice:

- Loss of consciousness
- Death
- Coma

Glucose Surge

MANAGING BLOOD GLUCOSE LEVELS

Your body typically controls your blood sugar levels by creating insulin, a hormone that enables your cells to utilize the blood sugar that is circulated in them.

Insulin is therefore the most significant factor in controlling blood sugar levels. To help prevent or postpone long-term, major health issues including heart disease, eyesight loss, and kidney disease, it's crucial to maintain your blood sugar levels as close to your target range as you can.

You might feel more energized and content by maintaining your target range. Your whole health and quality of life depend on you managing your blood sugar levels actively and purposefully.

Keeping your blood sugar levels within your goal range will help you prevent negative symptoms and health issues.

Maintaining healthy blood sugar levels can help you avoid negative symptoms and health issues while allowing you to feel your best and accomplish whatever it is that you set out to do in life.

What Are Some Ways To Treat Low Blood Glucose Level?

15-15 Rule

The "15-15 Rule," recommended by the American Diabetes Association, can be used by persons whose blood sugar levels are low (less than 70 mg/dL). It instructs them to eat 15 g of carbohydrates, wait 15 minutes, and then recheck their levels. Repeat until at least 70 mg/dL is reached if the reading is still low.

Given the lag time of continuous glucose monitors, it is advised that you check your blood sugar with a conventional glucometer instead. These foods have roughly 15 grams of carbohydrates:

1. ½ cup or 1 cup of juice or regular soda
2. 1 tablespoon of sugar, honey, or syrup
3. Gumdrops, jellybeans, or hard candies
4. 1 slice of bread
5. 1 small piece of fresh fruit
6. A cup of yogurt
7. ½ to 1 cup of skim milk.
8. Glucose tablets as indicated on the label
9. Glucose gel as indicated on the label

Keep the following in mind:
After eating, blood sugar levels take time to rise. Allow some time for the treatment to take effect. Following the 15-15 rule is beneficial.
Young children, especially newborns and toddlers, often require less than 15 grams of carbohydrates per day. Inquire with your doctor about how much your youngster requires.

Avoid eating both high-fat and high-fiber carbohydrates, such as chocolate and beans or lentils. Fiber and fat slow the rate at which sugar is absorbed.

When the weather is hot or you are traveling, check your blood sugar levels frequently.

How To Treat Severe Low Blood Glucose Level

An extremely low blood sugar reading is one that is below 55 mg/dL. It cannot be treated using the 15-15 rule. Depending on your symptoms, you might not even be able to monitor or treat your blood sugar on your own. Ascertain that your family, friends, and caregivers are well-aware of your low glucose level symptoms so that they can aid you with treatment if necessary.

Injectable glucagon is the most effective treatment for severely low blood sugar levels. A glucagon kit is available on prescription.

Consult your doctor to determine whether you need a kit. Ensure you understand when and how to utilize it.

Ensure that family members and anyone close to are aware of the place you store the glucagon kit and that they have received training on how to utilize it as well.

After getting a glucagon injection, it's crucial to call a doctor right away for emergency medical care. A glucagon injection usually causes a fainting (passing out) victim to regain consciousness within 15 minutes. One further dose should be administered if they don't awaken within 15 minutes of the initial injection. Upon awakening and being able to swallow, feed the person something that will release sugar quickly, such as fruit juice or a standard soft drink. Then, have them consume a long-acting source of sugar (a sandwich with meat or crackers and cheese).

Additionally, anybody who may come into contact with you frequently including friends, family, coworkers, teachers, coaches, and others must know how to check your blood sugar and treat severely low blood sugar as it develops.

After Low Blood Glucose

Once your blood sugar is back in the desired range, if your low blood sugar was mild (between 55 and 69 mg/dL), you can resume your regular activities. Your initial low blood sugar symptoms will be less obvious for 48 to 72 hours after you have them.

Check your blood sugar more frequently to prevent it from falling too low again, especially before engaging in physical activity, eating, or operating a motor vehicle.

Call your doctor right away for emergency medical care if you used glucagon due to a severe low (54 mg/dL or lower). Additionally, you should let your doctor know if you experience lows frequently, even if they are not severe. They could opt to change your diabetes plan.

If you continue to experience low blood sugar episodes, discuss your blood sugar, insulin, physical activity, and meal logs with your doctor. They may be able to detect patterns and prevent low glucose levels by adjusting the timing and amount of insulin you take, as well as your physical activity and meals.

What Are Some Ways To Treat High Blood Glucose Level?

Regular exercise

A healthy weight can be attained and maintained with regular exercise, which also increases insulin sensitivity. If your insulin sensitivity is increased, the available sugar in your bloodstream can be utilized more effectively by your cells. Exercise also improves your muscles' ability to use blood sugar for energy and contraction.

If you have difficulties controlling your blood sugar, consider testing it frequently before and after exercise. As a result, you'll be able to discover how you respond to various activities and avoid having too-high or too-low blood sugar levels.

Limit your carbs consumption

Your blood glucose levels are significantly impacted by the amount of carbohydrates you consume. Carbohydrates are converted by your body into sugars, primarily glucose. Following that, insulin assists your body in utilizing and storing it as energy. When you ingest too many carbohydrates or have problems with insulin function, this mechanism can break down and blood glucose levels can rise.

A low-carbohydrate diet lowers blood sugar levels and prevents blood sugar spikes. It's crucial to understand that low-carb and low-carbohydrate diets are not equivalent.

You can still have a few carbs while monitoring your blood sugar.

But choosing whole grains over processed grains and refined carbohydrates offers more nutritional benefits and lowers blood sugar levels.

Remain hydrated by drinking water

By consuming enough water, you might be able to keep your blood sugar levels in check. In addition to preventing dehydration, it helps the kidneys get rid of any extra sugar in the urine. Regular water intake may help the blood to become more hydrated, lower blood sugar levels, and reduce the risk of developing diabetes. Always keep in mind that water and other calorie-free beverages are the best. Products with added sugar should be avoided as they can raise blood sugar levels, lead to weight gain, and increase the risk of getting diabetes.

Develop portion control

Maintaining a healthy weight can be accomplished by portion control and calorie restriction.

Weight control, therefore, encourages normal blood glucose levels and has been demonstrated to lower the risk of acquiring type 2 diabetes. Keeping an eye on your serving amounts might help reduce blood sugar increases.The following are some helpful ideas for limiting portion sizes:

- Weigh and measure your servings.
- Use smaller plates
- Examine the portion sizes and food labels
- Eat slowly
- Keep a food journal

Consume foods with a low glycemic index

The glycemic index (GI) gauges how quickly your body consumes carbohydrates and how quickly they break down after digestion. This affects how quickly your blood sugar levels rise. According to the GI, which ranks foods from 0 to 100, foods are categorized as low, medium, or high GI. Low GI foods are those having a ranking of 55 or less. It has been shown that consuming low-GI meals in particular helps diabetics control their blood sugar levels.

For example, the following foods have a low to moderate GI:

- Bulgur
- Barley
- Unsweetened Greek yogurt
- Oats
- Beans
- Lentils
- Legumes
- Whole wheat pasta
- Non-starchy vegetables

Glucose Surge

DIABETES AND BLOOD GLUCOSE LEVELS

Keeping your blood glucose levels under control is an essential element of managing diabetes. That is due to the possibility of long-term problems from high blood sugar levels. When you have diabetes, your body is unable to produce any insulin or transport blood sugar into your cells.

High blood sugar or glucose levels result from this. One of the reasons blood sugar levels rise after meals is due to carbs in food. When you ingest foods containing carbohydrates, your body breaks those carbohydrates down into sugars.

These sugars circulate in the blood before reaching the cells. To meet the sugar at the cell, the pancreas, a tiny organ in the abdomen, releases the hormone insulin.

Insulin functions as a "bridge," enabling the transfer of sugar from the blood into the cell. Blood sugar levels decrease when the cell utilizes sugar as energy. The pancreas' ability to produce insulin, the cells' ability to use it, or both are compromised in people with diabetes.

What is Diabetes?

Diabetes is a condition in which your blood glucose levels are abnormally high. When you have diabetes, your body either produces insufficient insulin, uses it improperly, or both. A surplus of glucose is present in your blood but does not enter your cells. Over time, having excessive blood glucose levels can result in major health issues (diabetic complications). The various forms of diabetes and conditions connected to diabetes include:

1. **Type 1 diabetes** occurs when the body stops producing insulin.

2. **Type 2 diabetes**, which typically results from both insulin resistance and insufficient insulin production by the pancreas, is a metabolic disorder. Insulin resistance is present in those with type 2 diabetes. Although the body continues to manufacture insulin, it is unable to utilize it efficiently.

3. **Prediabetes** is when blood sugar levels are increased but not high enough to warrant a diabetes diagnosis.

4. **Gestational diabetes** is the term for diabetes that appears during the second or third trimester of pregnancy.

Therefore, it's crucial to maintain your blood glucose levels within your goal range if you have diabetes.

Blood Glucose Targets

Your blood glucose target is the range you strive to stay within if you have diabetes. Typical targets include:
- Before a meal: 80 to 130 mg/dL
- Two hours after the start of a meal: 180 mg/dL or less

When Should Blood Sugar Levels Be Checked?

If you have diabetes, you should probably check your blood glucose levels daily to make sure they are within the desired range. Some people may need to monitor their blood glucose levels numerous times during the day. Inquire with your doctor about how frequently you should check it. Among the alternatives are:
- After fasting (after waking or not eating for eight to twelve hours) or before meals
- Before and after meals to determine how the meal affected your blood sugar levels

- Before all meals, to determine how much insulin to inject
- At night

How Can Your Blood Glucose Levels Be Checked?

To measure your blood glucose levels, a blood sample is required. There are various ways to accomplish this at home.

1. Blood glucose monitor

The most popular tool for gauging blood sugar is a home glucose meter. The most popular kind of blood glucose monitor pricks your finger's side tip with a lancet to draw a tiny amount of blood. After that, you apply this drop of blood to a temporary test strip. The testing strip is then placed into an electronic blood glucose meter, which calculates the sample's glucose levels and displays a result on a digital readout.

2. Continuous glucose monitors

Another technique to assess your blood glucose levels is continuous glucose monitoring (CGM). The majority of CGM devices use a small sensor that is inserted beneath your skin. Your blood sugar level is measured every few minutes by the sensor. Your glucose level may fluctuate during the day and night, according to this test. The use of a CGM system is particularly beneficial for those who use insulin and experience low blood glucose issues.

What Measures Should You Take If Your Blood Glucose Is Too High?

Developing a treatment plan with your doctor is a good idea. You may be able to better manage your blood sugar levels by making dietary changes and other lifestyle adjustments, such as decreasing weight. Additionally, exercise can lower your blood glucose levels.

If your blood glucose levels are consistently high, tell your doctor.

This could entail changing your diabetic treatment regimen or using regular medication. It's crucial to work with your doctor to control your blood sugar levels. Serious consequences including diabetic neuropathy or renal failure might result from persistently high levels.

Monitor your blood sugar levels
You can manage your blood glucose levels more effectively by monitoring them. This can be done at home with a glucometer, also known as a portable blood glucose meter. You can discuss this option with your doctor.
You can assess whether you need to change your diet or medicine by keeping track. Additionally, it teaches you about how your body responds to certain foods.
Consider monitoring your levels frequently throughout the day and keeping a note of the results. Additionally, monitoring your blood sugar in pairs may be more beneficial, such as before and after a workout or before and two hours after a meal.

If a meal raises your blood sugar, this can help you determine whether you should alter it slightly rather than completely stop eating it.

Medication

Depending on your needs, doctors could add drugs to your regimen. Metformin is typically the first drug prescribed to persons with type 2 diabetes. Diabetes drugs come in a wide variety and have various mechanisms of action.

Insulin

One method to swiftly lower your blood sugar levels is to inject insulin. To control blood glucose levels, people with type 1 diabetes must inject insulin several times daily. Your physician will establish your dosage and go over the best timing for injection with you.

Sleep well enough

A healthy lifestyle depends on getting enough sleep, which feels great. In actuality, poor sleeping patterns and a lack of sleep can have an impact on insulin sensitivity and blood sugar levels, raising the risk of type 2 diabetes. They may also stimulate the appetite and encourage weight gain. Cortisol levels also increase as a result of sleep loss. As previously mentioned, cortisol is a key hormone in the regulation of blood sugar. Try some of these things in order to have a better night's sleep:

- Maintain a sleeping pattern
- Avoid consuming coffee and alcohol in the evening
- Limit your naps in the afternoon
- Engage in regular exercise
- Reduce your screen time before night
- Create a nighttime routine
- When going to bed, take a warm bath or shower
- Avoid working in your bedroom

Make a meal plan

Your glucose levels can be significantly impacted by the things you eat. Include lean proteins, fiber-rich foods, and nutritious carbohydrates in your diet.

Suitable carbs consist of vegetables, fruits, whole grains and legumes such as beans.

When eating meals and snacks, be mindful of how many good carbohydrates you consume. To slow digestion and prevent blood sugar rises, add protein and fat.

It's crucial to include healthy fats in a diabetes diet. Monounsaturated and polyunsaturated fats should be prioritized above saturated and trans fats, according to the ADA.

Healthy fats help reduce a person's cholesterol levels, heart disease risk, and other diabetes-related issues. Among the options are: oily fish, nuts, seeds, avocados, olives, and olive oil.

Diabetes patients should avoid foods and beverages that raise blood sugar levels. These are some examples: highly refined carbs such as white bread and pasta, high sugar content foods such as candies and sugary soft drinks.

Diabetes patients should also avoid meals that increase the risk of cardiovascular disease.

These are some examples: saturated and trans-fat-rich foods, foods high in sodium and alcohol.

The first step in treating your diabetes is to regularly check your blood glucose levels. Knowing your numbers will also enable you to tell your doctor about any potential adjustments to your treatment regimen.

You should be able to maintain normal glucose levels by eating a balanced diet, exercising, and taking your medications as directed. If you're unsure of how to take drugs or need assistance creating a diet or exercise plan, speak with your doctor.

FOOD AND BLOOD GLUCOSE LEVELS

Numerous foods may reduce blood sugar, but some may do it more quickly. Although other factors that affect blood sugar control include body weight, activity, stress, and genetics, maintaining a nutritious diet is essential for blood sugar control. While some foods, such as those that are high in added sugar and refined carbohydrates, might cause blood sugar fluctuations, other foods can improve blood sugar management while enhancing general health.

For persons who want to control their blood sugar levels, foods with low or medium GI scores are preferable. People can also pair foods with low and high GI ratings in order to make a meal balanced. Researchers contend that low GI eating habits can enhance a person's health.

According to research, long-term low GI dietary patterns can enhance a person's blood sugar response. The greatest foods and drinks for diabetics are those that the body absorbs slowly because they prevent blood sugar spikes and troughs. One strategy for lowering or managing blood sugar levels is to choose foods with a low glycemic index (GI).

The GI measures the impact of various foods on blood sugar levels. The foods listed below are some of the best for people trying to keep their blood sugar levels in check.

1. Fruits

Most fruits, except for melons and pineapples, have low GI ratings of 55 or lower. This is because most fresh fruits have a lot of water and fiber to counteract the fructose, a sugar that is present naturally in them. Fruits' GI scores rise as they ripen, though. Because the fibrous skins and seeds are removed during juicing, fruit liquids also have extremely high GI scores. Fresh fruit is therefore preferred.

Fruits to consume
- apples
- peaches
- raspberries
- blueberries
- grapefruit
- grapes
- plums
- strawberries
- apricots
- avocadoes

Fruits to be consumed in moderation
dates
- overripe bananas
- dried fruit
- watermelon
- pineapple fruit juice

2. Oat bran and Oatmeal

Oats have a GI score of 55 or below, which makes them less prone to trigger blood sugar spikes and dips.

Additionally, oats include -glucan, which can increase insulin sensitivity, aid maintain glycemic control, and reduce blood lipids (fats) as well as decrease glucose and insulin responses after meals.

Good ways to eat oats include rolled oats and stone-ground oats. Oat products such as instant oats, cereal bars and processed oats should be limited.

3. Fatty fish

Due to the lack of carbohydrates in fish and other meats, GI ratings are not available for these foods. However, compared to other meats, eating fish that is rich in the omega-3 fatty acids docosahexaenoic acid and eicosapentaenoic acid may help manage or prevent diabetes.

The ability to better regulate blood sugar has been linked to a high intake of fatty fish like salmon and sardines.

Other fish products to consume are anchovies, cod, haddock, herring, pollock, saithe and fish oil capsules.

Bigeye tuna, swordfish, tilefish, king mackerel, and marlin shark are among the fish to be limited.

4. Nuts

Nuts are incredibly high in dietary fiber and have GI scores of 55 or less. Additionally, nuts are rich in plant proteins, unsaturated fatty acids, antioxidants, vitamins, and phytochemicals like flavonoids, magnesium, and potassium.

Nuts should ideally be consumed as whole and unprocessed as feasible. The GI ratings of coated or flavored nuts are greater than those of unflavored nuts. Raw almonds, raw cashews, raw walnuts, raw pecans, other tree nuts, raw peanuts, peanut butter, and sunflower seeds are all edible nut products. Cashews, macadamia nuts, roasted or salted nuts, and candied nuts are nuts with higher GI scores.

5. Okra

A fruit that is frequently utilized as a vegetable is okra. It contains a lot of polysaccharides and blood sugar-lowering flavonoid antioxidants.

Okra seeds' powerful blood sugar-lowering abilities make them a potential asset as a natural diabetes treatment. It has been discovered that the main polysaccharide in okra, rhamnogalacturonan, has potent anti-diabetic properties. Okra also contains the flavonoids isoquercitrin and quercetin which work by inhibiting specific enzymes to lower blood sugar.

6. Legumes

Beans, peas, chickpeas, and lentils are examples of legumes with very low GI ratings. Even less appealing baked beans still have a medium GI grade. Legumes high in nutrients can help maintain appropriate blood sugar levels. They contain protein, fiber, and complex carbs.

The legumes such as black beans, pinto beans, green beans, lima beans, navy beans, black-eyed peas, chickpeas, lentils, snow peas, and hummus can all be consumed.

7. Seafood

A valuable source of protein, good fats, vitamins, minerals, and antioxidants that may help control blood sugar levels is seafood, which includes fish and shellfish. Protein is crucial for controlling blood sugar. It promotes sluggish digestion, reduces blood sugar surges after meals, and heightens feelings of satiety.

Additionally, it could aid in the reduction of extra body fat and overeating, two factors that are crucial for maintaining normal blood sugar levels.

8. Garlic

Garlic is often used in traditional treatments for diabetes and a variety of other ailments. Garlic components may help lower blood sugar by enhancing insulin sensitivity and secretion.

How to incorporate garlic into your diet
- eating it raw
- slicing it and adding it to dips, savory spreads, and salad dressings
- sauteing it with vegetables

- adding it to cooked meals
- garlic capsules

9. Yogurt

Consuming plain yogurt daily may lower the chance of developing type 2 diabetes. Plain yogurt has a low GI. The GI of most unsweetened yogurts is 50 or lower. It is advisable to avoid sweetened or flavored yogurts, which typically contain far too much sugar for someone trying to control their blood sugar levels. Greek yogurt is a nutritious option in addition to yogurt without sugar.

10. Eggs

Eggs are a rich source of protein, healthy fats, vitamins, minerals, and antioxidants. Some research has connected egg eating to better blood sugar management.

11. Bread

A variety of bread can raise blood sugar levels and have high GI ratings. Therefore, many are better avoided by those who have diabetes.

However, eating foods made from whole grains has been linked to a reduced incidence of type 2 diabetes. Some breads are regarded as a healthy whole-grain food source.

Whole wheat bread, particularly stone ground, wheat bread, pumpernickel, spelt, rye, and rice bread produced with ancient grains like emmer and einkorn, as well as bread made from less-processed grains, are all recommended. Fruit bread, raisin toast, white bread, bagels, and other bread prepared with refined or finely ground grains should be avoided.

A balanced food pattern is crucial for proper blood sugar management. Whether you have prediabetes or diabetes or want to lessen your risk of acquiring these disorders, consuming the items listed above as part of a balanced diet may help lower your blood sugar levels.

However, bear in mind that your entire nutritional consumption, as well as characteristics like your activity level and body weight, are the most crucial when it comes to

improving blood sugar regulation and protecting
against chronic disease.

EXERCISE AND BLOOD GLUCOSE LEVELS

Exercising is one of the most popular blood sugar-lowering recommendations from doctors. However, they also assert that exercise raises blood sugar levels. Which of the following is true?

Both but controlling your metabolic health requires that you have a solid understanding of why this is the case. If you have prediabetes or a strong family history of diabetes, it's very crucial. This is because exercise can help stop or delay the onset of type 2 diabetes, making prediabetes a reversible condition!

Each person may experience alterations in glucose levels differently. Your diet, general health, and the type, length, and intensity of your physical exercise can all have an impact on the outcome.

Depending on the kind, length, and level of physical activity you engage in as well as your nutrition and general state of health, the outcome may vary. The link between exercise and blood sugar is therefore complicated.

Finding a signal in the noise that will direct you toward controlling your blood sugar levels is the aim. Doing so will allow you to benefit from having a healthy metabolism. Jumping right into the science is the easiest approach to comprehending the connection between exercise and blood sugar.

Are Your Glucose Levels Affected by Exercise?

Exercise can lower blood sugar levels for up to 24 hours (or more), according to the American Diabetes Association.

Your muscle cells utilize the insulin that is available to them more effectively, increasing your insulin sensitivity (more on this later).

Compared to when they are at rest, your muscles utilize more glucose when they are working.

This increased blood sugar absorption by your muscles naturally reduces blood sugar levels.

How Exercise Affects Glucose Instantly

Your body uses glucose and fat as energy sources when you work out. The intensity of your workout and the type of fuel your body is using will both have an impact on how your blood sugar changes while you're working out. Running or relaxed swimming are examples of steady-state cardio sports that don't require your body to produce sudden bursts of energy. Because it obtains more of its energy from fat in these circumstances, your blood sugar will often remain stable or drop.

Your body releases an adrenaline rush when you perform higher-intensity exercises like HIIT(high-intensity interval training), weight training, and sprinting. Your body releases glucose from your liver, raising your blood sugar levels to make sure you have adequate energy available for this.

Simply put, supply and demand are used by your body when you exercise. It lacks the energy supply needed to fuel your workout when performing high-intensity exercises. As a result, it releases glucose, instantly supplying the energy needed to fuel your workout while also generating a brief increase in blood sugar. Your body has enough energy stored for the activity to match the demand, thus during low-intensity exercise, blood glucose levels usually remain stable or even drop.

How Exercise Affects Glucose Over Time

Nothing could be more clear-cut. The long-term benefits of exercise for blood sugar levels outweigh the occasional glucose increase. All forms of exercise enhance insulin sensitivity and blood sugar regulation, according to the American College of Sports Medicine and the American Diabetes Association.

How Come Exercise Is So Vital For Your Glucose Levels?

Blood glucose remains higher than it would be in the absence of exercise. High blood sugar damages blood vessels in a variety of ways that result in several health problems, including retinal damage, which can result in blindness.

Maintaining healthy blood glucose levels with exercise. Blood vessel damage is prevented by normal blood glucose levels.

Because persons with diabetes have a two to four times higher risk of developing cardiovascular disease than those without the disease, not exercising leads to poorer levels of cardiovascular fitness, which can be problematic. This elevated risk is a result of some medical conditions, such as high blood pressure, high cholesterol, and obesity.

Having poor cardiovascular health in people with diabetes is highly correlated with a higher risk of death from any cause.

What Exercises Are Beneficial for Blood Glucose Levels?

Exercise and blood sugar levels have a beneficial association. That much is obvious. However, this relationship can vary based on your exercise habits and whether you have diabetes.

Your blood sugar levels may benefit from engaging in these different types of exercise.

1. Strength Training

Exercises for increasing muscle strength, mass, and endurance in strength training include weightlifting (free or machine), bodyweight exercises, and resistance bands.

It is aerobic to do strength training. Your body uses glucose as its primary source of energy while you exercise anaerobically. Oxygen is not required for glucose breakdown. You get short-term high energy surges from doing this. Anaerobic exercise helps with blood sugar regulation and insulin sensitivity, according to the American Diabetes Association.

Strength training also contributes to our ability to gain lean muscle mass. Only the liver and skeletal muscle can store glycogen, that glucose-holding compartment we briefly discussed before. Therefore, the potential capacity of your body to store incoming glucose increases as muscle mass does. This results in lower and better managed blood glucose levels.

2. Walking

Never underestimate the benefits a stroll around the park may have on your well-being. Your breathing and heart rate both get a little faster when you're walking. Your muscles will be encouraged to use more glucose as a result, which will assist control your blood sugar levels. Keep in mind that exercise doesn't have to be strenuous to have an effect. Walking is a good exercise to help you manage your blood sugar levels. Therefore, even a short walk after dinner can significantly improve your metabolic health.

3. Stability

Flexibility and balance are enhanced by stability exercises. Yoga, tai chi, stretching, and balance exercises fall under this category. These actions can undoubtedly help with blood sugar regulation.

4. Swimming

Swimming is a fantastic cardiovascular exercise for people with type 2 diabetes since it is easy on the joints.

5. Running

You can progress from walking quickly to running with the right instruction and the approval of your doctor. The risk of high blood pressure, high blood sugar, and high cholesterol has been found to be lower while engaging in this faster-paced activity.

6. Cycling

Regular riding can enhance your balance and posture as well as your heart and lung health. But to get started, you don't need a pricey fitness bike. You may either try a stationary cycle at your neighborhood gym or grab an old bike and head outside. Additionally, studies indicate that cycling can enhance the health of diabetics.

7. High-intensity interval training

You can alternate between short periods of high-intensity exercises and longer periods of lower-intensity movements when you do HIIT (high-intensity interval training). It can be added to a variety of workouts, including cycling and running. HIIT may help your Type 2 diabetes by lowering your fasting blood sugar.

8. Dancing

Your exercise program may become more enjoyable if you incorporate dance. Dancing is a heart-healthy activity that also helps with blood sugar control and fitness.

What Exercises Affect Blood Glucose Levels Negatively?

Exercise clearly has a good impact on blood sugar regulation. Do you need to weigh any drawbacks, though? Simply said, not really. To exercise safely, there are a few considerations to bear in mind. All forms of exercise are advantageous if you are in good health and don't have any underlying illnesses or worries. This is true. To improve your performance and metabolic health, there are a few things to watch out for. High-intensity exercise can result in a blood sugar rise, as previously discussed. All forms of exercise are advantageous if you are in good health and don't have any underlying illnesses or worries.

There are a few things to watch out for to improve your metabolic health and performance. As previously indicated, intense exercise can create a blood sugar spike, so aim to limit one that exceeds 180 mg/dL. This is due to the possibility of blood vessel damage caused by abnormally high glucose surges like this.

You can avoid blood sugar rises once you are aware of how your body responds to activity. If you do discover that you experience a significant glycemic response to exercise, be mindful of your pre-workout calorie, fluid, and electrolyte consumption. In situations like these, employing a continuous glucose monitor for training and fitness may be beneficial. Because extremely high glucose surges like these have the potential to harm blood vessels.

To control your blood sugar levels both during and after exercise, consider the following advice:

- Check your blood sugar levels before, during, and after working out to ensure that you exercise safely.
- Learn to recognize trends and become familiar with your regular ranges.
- Before exercising, eat a modest snack that combines fat, protein, and carbohydrates.
- Keep yourself hydrated when working out.

- After working out, try grabbing a carb-based snack to eat right away if your blood sugar levels dip.

For Those With Diabetes

All sorts of exercise are quite useful if you have diabetes. But there are other safety measures to observe when working out. Additionally, if you wish to begin a new or particularly rigorous fitness regimen, you should consult a doctor.

If your blood sugar is too high or too low, avoid exercising.

Never work out if your blood sugar is too high or too low before you begin. This is due to the possibility that it will make you feel sick and further raise or reduce your blood sugar levels.

Exercise can be risky if your blood sugar is more than 250 mg/dL (13.9 mmol/L). Prioritize lowering your blood sugar levels before a workout.

Your blood sugar levels during exercise will soar if you have high glucose levels and no insulin in your system. Additionally, you run the danger of developing diabetic ketoacidosis, a potentially fatal condition in which your body starts metabolizing fat too quickly.

A blood sugar level between 100 and 250 mg/dL (5.6 to 13.9 mmol/L) is generally considered safe for the majority of diabetics to exercise. An excessive glucose increase can also be brought on by high-intensity workouts. You should be especially mindful of this if you have diabetes, particularly type 1 diabetes, or use insulin treatment.

When a person has type 1 diabetes, the body is unable to produce more insulin to counteract an increase in blood sugar. Therefore, it's critical to test glucose levels more frequently while engaging in vigorous exercise, maintain them within safe ranges, and modify insulin dosages as necessary.

It may not be safe for you to exercise if you have diabetes and your blood sugar levels are below 70 mg/dL (3.9 mmol/L). Consider consuming a little snack to raise your blood sugar levels, then check them again before working out.

When exercising, low blood sugar can also be a problem, especially if you work out for a long time. If you're lengthening or intensifying your workout regimen, it's definitely something to keep in mind.

The 15:15 rule should be followed if you develop hypoglycemia while exercising.

How Should You Monitor Your Blood Glucose Levels While Working Out?

You may examine your body's reaction by checking your blood sugar levels before, during, and after exercise. You may exercise safely, perform at your peak, and achieve your health goals by being aware of how your blood glucose levels change when you're working out.

Using a continuous glucose monitor (CGM) while exercising, such as weightlifting or jogging, is one approach to tracking your blood sugar in real time. Your smartphone app will instantly provide you with access to your real-time glucose readings after you simply scan the sensor.

This enables you to observe how your blood sugar levels change in response to particular foods, stress, or exercise. Based on the information provided by your own body, you may then alter your lifestyle for the better.

Glucose Surge

TECHNOLOGY AND BLOOD GLUCOSE LEVELS

Diabetes glucose management primarily aims to protect persons with diabetes from consequences like eye, kidney, and nerve issues as well as to ensure that they do not have dangerously high or low blood sugar levels.

Innovative technology has led to improvements in the treatment of diabetes over time. Various technologies are currently available that can assist you in managing your diabetes. When your healthcare provider discusses diabetes technology, they typically mean equipment that makes it easier for you to take insulin or equipment that measures your blood sugar levels.

The optimal glucose management solution will change as technology develops and depending on your individual tastes.

Which solution is best for you should be discussed with your doctor. Options may be made simpler to fit your lifestyle if you are aware of the differences between each.

Continuous glucose monitoring (CGM) is a wearable gadget that continuously monitors glucose levels. The amount of glucose present in the fluid separating cells, or interstitial glucose, is measured by a sensor positioned beneath the skin of the arm or belly. It may be placed on the buttocks in younger individuals.

It is made to continuously monitor your blood glucose levels and offers you a glimpse of them at any given moment.

Real-time monitoring of your glucose levels throughout the day can provide you insight into where your blood sugar is and where it is heading, allowing you to identify patterns and make appropriate adjustments to better balance your blood glucose. If you have type 2 diabetes, take insulin, experience significant blood sugar swings, suffer hypoglycemia, or simply want more information about blood sugar, a continuous glucose monitor may be beneficial to you. Some noteworthy features are:

- Alarms warning you when your blood sugar levels are high or low
- The capability of monitoring one's diet, exercise, and medicine intake
- Data that is readily downloadable and accessible on a computer or smartphone

Insulin Pump

A computerized gadget linked to the body called an insulin pump enables continuous insulin delivery. Some pumps can be attached with a catheter and others without tubing. A third choice is a disposable pump patch that does not need a catheter or tubing. Throughout the day, the pump releases insulin into the bloodstream as needed.

The pump assists users in preventing daily blood sugar peaks and valleys, which maintains steady insulin levels. The automatic delivery of insulin throughout the day makes it possible to maintain tighter blood sugar control. Avoiding significant glucose changes is helpful. The quantity of insulin required to maintain normal blood sugar levels is known as the basal amount, and the pump is programmed to administer this amount. While the pump automatically administers insulin, it can also be used manually to administer insulin as needed. Before eating, fast-acting insulin can be given to lower blood sugar levels.

CGM-Insulin Pumps

Better diabetes management is promoted by pairing a CGM with an insulin pump. The insulin pump can be set up for the day using the data collected by the CGM. By lowering the risk of high or low blood sugar, using both devices at once has been found to help manage diabetes significantly.

Glucometers

A glucometer, also called a blood glucose monitor, is a tiny instrument that gauges a person's blood sugar levels using a tiny blood sample. These meters can only provide a person with their current blood sugar readings. The instrument makes use of a blood sample that you obtain by pinching your finger. The blood is then collected on a tiny sensory tab, which is subsequently inserted into the meter. A common monitoring tool in the management of diabetes is the glucometer.

Insulin Pens

A tool that contains insulin is called an insulin pen. The pen contains insulin vials or cartridges that can be manually administered using a disposable needle. They provide users with the option to administer their insulin shots wherever they are, thus those who are more mobile tend to utilize them. Two types of insulin pens exist:

- Disposable
- Reusable

Disposable

Insulin cartilage is found in disposable pens, which are discarded after they are empty.

Reusable

Once the ink runs out, reusable pens can be refilled with fresh cartridges. You discard the used ink cartridge and preserve the pen. Reusable smart device pens can measure dosages and give crucial information for managing diabetes when used with a companion app. Additionally, smart insulin pens can

- determine the required dose based on the current glucose levels.
- keep a record of your doses, including when the previous dose was given and the dosage amount.
- set a reminder for you to take your next dose.
- inform you when to change the insulin cartridge
- send details about your diabetes to your doctor so they can easily determine where you stand with your management.

Phone applications

Apps for smartphones are frequently used to support managing diabetes. They keep tabs on their diet, activity, blood sugar levels, medicine, and carbohydrate intake.

Although useful, the applications must be used in conjunction with a different monitoring device if you want to keep track of your blood glucose levels. The best app depends largely on what you want to track because there are several to select from.

Telemedicine

Telemedicine is the practice of giving medical care over the phone or the internet. It is frequently utilized when being in close proximity to your healthcare professional is not necessary.

People who receive this sort of healthcare receive continuing assistance in controlling their diabetes by helping them monitor their treatment programs, become familiar with new treatment alternatives, and undergo screenings for any complications the condition may have.

The ability to monitor blood glucose levels and control diabetes is now more accessible than ever thanks to technological advancements. A person can efficiently maintain track of their blood sugar levels with the help of a variety of digital alternatives, including smart insulin pens, glucose monitoring devices, and apps.

You can live a more liberated life and control your diabetes much more easily with the help of technology. Technology can connect you to others in some circumstances. Although it doesn't directly monitor your diabetes, doing so can still be beneficial in helping you manage it.

STRESS AND BLOOD GLUCOSE LEVELS

The effects of stress on the body, whether mental or physical, can vary widely. One of the health effects it might have is a spike in blood sugar.

The body produces more cortisol, the main stress hormone, when it is subjected to high amounts of chronic stress. The body secretes less insulin when there is an increase in blood cortisol levels. Insulin aids in bringing sugar from the bloodstream into cells, where it is used as fuel. More sugar lingers in the bloodstream and blood sugar levels become unbalanced without the normal insulin release. Stress has the potential to affect blood sugar levels both directly and indirectly. Additionally, depending on the type of diabetes a person has, the effects can change. Stress-related behaviors, such as emotional overeating of refined carbohydrates or foods with a lot of added sugar, can result in high blood sugar levels. Additionally, people could neglect to exercise or take their prescribed prescriptions on time. These elements may all contribute to increased blood sugar levels since stress has the power to alter good behaviors.

Stress has the potential to both raise and lower blood sugar levels in people with type 1 diabetes. Chronic stress can result in adrenal exhaustion syndrome when it reduces blood sugar levels. Long-term stress exposure depletes the adrenal glands, resulting in low cortisol levels and adrenal fatigue.

A hormonal imbalance that affects the hormones responsible for controlling blood sugar levels can occur in people with type 1 diabetes because of the underproduction of certain hormones, such as cortisol.

High levels of stress can raise blood sugar levels in patients with type 2 diabetes. Body tissues become less responsive to insulin when there is a high quantity of cortisol in the body. As a result, there is more blood sugar available in the blood. When this occurs, blood sugar levels become unbalanced and may increase to hazardous levels, particularly if untreated.

How To Control Your Stress Levels

Some types of stress are uncontrollable, especially if they don't occur frequently, like a single traumatic occurrence or an unintentional injury. Other forms of stress, such as caring for family members, workplace pressures, or any other regular stressful situations, are likely to last permanently or semi-permanently. It is important to manage these stressful situations as best you can.

You can proactively prepare for this by doing so. This entails organizing your time, reading self-help literature, or reducing the source of stress as much as you can, in addition to being ready for life's usual stressors. Meditation and other calming practices like yoga have also been shown to lower stress levels.

Additionally, you should refrain from engaging in unhealthy habits like binge eating. It might feel reassuring at the time, but it won't help you deal with the stress you're under.

For those with diabetes, setting attainable goals can significantly reduce stress. Setting a goal of walking for at least half an hour every day on particular days of the week will be much more doable than concentrating on a big and ambiguous objective like losing weight.

Nobody can completely avoid stress because it is a natural part of life. This is why it's crucial to safeguard yourself against the effects of stress by putting a plan in place to help handle both stressful events and spikes or declines in blood sugar levels. Making your health the top priority when under stress might be challenging, but it's not impossible to accomplish.

CONCLUSION

One of your body's most vital molecules, glucose gives your cells the majority of the energy they require to operate. A disruption in our glucose levels can cause issues to appear almost anywhere in our body, including the skin, brain, organs, and neurological system. This is because it impacts every cell in our bodies. It can interfere with hormones like insulin and cause further disorders.

Managing glucose problems early on is easier, as it is with many other medical diseases. Additionally, to maintain your body functioning at its peak, healthy glucose levels are imperative. It's critical to know your blood glucose levels because having readings that are either too high or too low might negatively impact your overall health.

You can avoid negative symptoms and health issues by avoiding too-high or too-low blood sugar levels, and maintaining your goal range can help you feel your best.

A healthy, balanced diet, stress management through relaxation techniques, and exercise are all components of prevention and treatment regimens that can help you control your blood sugar levels. But for some, this isn't sufficient.

Diabetes patients may struggle to maintain normal, consistent glucose levels. Monitoring your glucose levels carefully is an efficient strategy to help prevent complications if you have diabetes. Additionally, keeping a daily journal enables you to change your diet and prescriptions as needed to better control your blood sugar levels.

The best course of action is to develop a treatment plan with your healthcare physician because optimum blood sugar levels might differ significantly from person to person. You can decide how to manage your levels most effectively together.

 If you need assistance creating a diet or exercise plan or if you have questions about how to take drugs, you can also discuss these issues with your doctor.
Although managing your diabetes might be difficult, it is worth the effort.